The Endomorph Meal Plan and Exercise for Seniors

Balancing Diet and Exercise for Healthy Aging

Rosalee Casper

Table of Contents

Welcome to Your Endomorph Journey

Aging gracefully and maintaining optimal health is a journey that requires understanding and embracing your unique body type. As a senior with an endomorphic body type, you may have noticed that your body responds differently to diet and exercise compared to others. Endomorphs often have a higher propensity for storing fat, particularly around the midsection, and may find it more challenging to lose weight. However, this doesn't mean achieving your health and fitness goals is out of reach. In fact, with the right approach, you can unlock your full potential and enjoy a vibrant, healthy life.

This book is designed to guide you through every step of your journey. We'll delve into the science behind your body type, explore tailored nutrition and exercise plans, and provide practical tips to help you stay motivated and on track. Whether you're looking to lose weight, build strength, or simply improve your overall well-being, understanding your endomorphic body type is the key to success.

The first step in this journey is to embrace your endomorph identity. Recognize that your body type is not a limitation but a guide to what works best for you. Accepting and understanding your natural predispositions allows you to make informed decisions about your diet and exercise routines. This acceptance is not about settling for less but about optimizing your health by working with your body's natural tendencies.

One size does not fit all, especially when it comes to health and fitness. What works for others may not work for endomorphs. Tailoring your nutrition and exercise regimen to fit your body type can significantly enhance your results. This book will provide you with detailed guidelines and practical advice on how to adapt your lifestyle to suit your endomorphic needs.

Before diving into the specifics of diet and exercise, it's essential to set realistic and achievable goals. Understand that progress may be gradual, but every step forward is a victory. Set both short-term and long-term goals to keep yourself motivated and on track. For example, aim to lose a certain amount of weight each month, increase your strength over time, or simply improve your energy levels and overall well-being.

Embarking on this journey is much easier when you have a support system. Share your goals with family and friends, and consider joining a community of like-minded individuals who can offer encouragement and advice. Remember, you are not alone in this journey, and having a support system can make a significant difference in your success.

As you read through this book, keep an open mind and be patient with yourself. Change doesn't happen overnight, but with dedication and the right strategies, you can achieve a healthier, happier life. Welcome to your endomorph journey – let's take the first step together.

Introduction

As you embark on this journey to better health and fitness, it's essential to understand the unique characteristics of your endomorphic body type. This knowledge will empower you to make informed decisions about your diet and exercise routines, helping you achieve your goals more effectively. Let's explore the specific traits of the endomorph body type and how they impact your health and wellness.

Characteristics of the Endomorph Body Type

Endomorphs typically have a higher percentage of body fat, especially around the abdomen, hips, and thighs. This body type is often characterized by a larger bone structure and a softer, rounder physique. Common traits of endomorphs include:

- Slower Metabolism: Endomorphs tend to have a slower metabolic rate, which means they burn calories more slowly. This can make weight loss more challenging, as the body stores excess calories as fat more readily.

- Higher Fat Storage: Endomorphs are prone to storing fat, particularly in the lower body. This tendency can be frustrating, but understanding it allows you to tailor your diet and exercise to combat this trait.

- Muscle Development: While endomorphs may find it easier to gain fat, they also have a natural ability to build muscle. With the right exercise regimen, you can harness this potential to improve your body composition and boost your metabolism.

- Insulin Sensitivity: Endomorphs are often more sensitive to insulin, a hormone that regulates blood sugar levels. This sensitivity can lead to higher fat storage when consuming carbohydrates, so managing carbohydrate intake is crucial.

The Science Behind Your Body Type

Understanding the science behind your body type involves recognizing how your metabolism and hormones affect your weight and health. Endomorphs typically have a lower basal metabolic rate (BMR), which means they require fewer calories to maintain their weight. Additionally, endomorphs often experience greater fluctuations in blood sugar levels, which can impact energy levels and hunger.

Hormonal Influences

Several hormones play a significant role in the endomorph body type:

- Insulin: As mentioned earlier, endomorphs are often more insulin-sensitive. Insulin helps cells absorb glucose from the bloodstream. However, high levels of insulin can lead to increased fat storage. Managing carbohydrate intake and focusing on low-glycemic foods can help regulate insulin levels.
- Leptin: This hormone regulates hunger and energy balance. Endomorphs may have higher levels of leptin but can also be leptin-resistant, meaning their brains don't receive the signal to stop eating. Eating a balanced diet and incorporating regular physical activity can help improve leptin sensitivity.
- Cortisol: Known as the stress hormone, cortisol can contribute to fat storage, especially in the abdominal area. Managing stress through relaxation techniques, adequate sleep, and physical activity is essential for endomorphs.

Chapter 2: Nutritional Foundations for Endomorph Seniors

Adopting the right diet is essential for managing weight, optimizing health, and boosting energy levels, especially for endomorphic seniors. The endomorph diet is designed to cater specifically to the metabolic and physiological characteristics of individuals with an endomorphic body type. By understanding and implementing this diet, you can better manage your weight, improve your metabolic health, and enhance your overall well-being.

The Basics of the Endomorph Diet

The endomorph diet emphasizes a balanced intake of macronutrients—proteins, fats, and carbohydrates—tailored to the unique needs of endomorphs. Here are the foundational principles of the diet:

- Higher Protein Intake: Proteins are crucial for muscle maintenance and repair, especially as muscle mass naturally declines with age. A higher protein intake helps boost metabolism through the thermi

- c effect of food, where more energy is required to digest and metabolize proteins.
- Moderate Fat Intake: Healthy fats are important for maintaining energy levels and supporting cell function. Incorporate sources of monounsaturated and polyunsaturated fats, such as avocados, nuts, seeds, and olive oil, while limiting saturated fats.
- Lower Carbohydrate Intake: Since endomorphs tend to be more sensitive to insulin, controlling carbohydrate intake is vital. Focus on complex carbohydrates that have a low glycemic index to avoid spikes in blood sugar levels.

Meal Timing and Frequency

Endomorphs benefit from eating smaller, more frequent meals throughout the day. This approach helps regulate blood sugar levels and prevents overeating. Aim for three main meals and two to three small snacks, ensuring that each meal contains a balance of proteins, fats, and carbohydrates.

Foods to Avoid

To optimize the endomorph diet, it's important to limit or avoid certain foods that can hinder progress:

- Refined Sugars: Avoid sweets, sugary beverages, and desserts that cause spikes in blood sugar levels.
- Processed Foods: Steer clear of highly processed foods like chips, fast food, and pre-packaged meals, which are often high in unhealthy fats, sugars, and sodium.
- Refined Carbohydrates: Limit intake of white bread, pasta, and rice, which can lead to quick spikes and crashes in blood sugar.
- High-Sodium Foods: Reduce consumption of salty snacks, canned soups, and processed meats to avoid water retention and bloating.

Supplements

While a balanced diet should provide most nutrients, certain supplements can support the health of endomorph seniors:

- Omega-3 Fatty Acids: For heart health and inflammation reduction.
- Vitamin D: Especially important for bone health and immune function, as older adults may have lower levels.
- Magnesium: Supports muscle and nerve function, and can aid in relaxation and sleep.

- Probiotics: For digestive health, especially if you experience gastrointestinal issues.

Macronutrients: Balancing Carbohydrates, Proteins, and Fats

Balancing macronutrients—carbohydrates, proteins, and fats—is essential for maintaining optimal health and achieving your fitness goals as an endomorphic senior. Each macronutrient plays a unique role in your body, and understanding how to balance them can help you manage your weight, support muscle health, and maintain energy levels. In this sub-chapter, we will explore the functions of each macronutrient, recommended ratios for endomorphs, and practical tips for incorporating them into your diet.

Understanding Macronutrients

1. Carbohydrates

- Function: Carbohydrates are the body's primary source of energy. They are broken down into glucose, which fuels your brain, muscles, and other tissues.
- Types: Carbohydrates can be classified into simple and complex carbs. Simple carbs, found in sugary

foods and drinks, are quickly digested and can cause blood sugar spikes. Complex carbs, found in whole grains, vegetables, and legumes, are digested more slowly, providing sustained energy and helping to regulate blood sugar levels.

- Sources: Whole grains (quinoa, oats, brown rice), vegetables (especially non-starchy varieties like leafy greens, broccoli), fruits (berries, apples), and legumes.

2. Proteins

- Function: Proteins are essential for building and repairing tissues, producing enzymes and hormones, and supporting immune function. They also play a critical role in muscle maintenance and growth, which is particularly important for seniors to counteract age-related muscle loss.
- Sources: Lean meats (chicken, turkey), fish (salmon, tuna), eggs, dairy products (Greek yogurt, cottage cheese), legumes (beans, lentils), and plant-based proteins (tofu, tempeh).

3. Fats

- Function: Fats provide a concentrated source of energy, support cell structure and function, and aid in the absorption of fat-soluble vitamins (A, D, E, K). Healthy fats are crucial for brain health and reducing inflammation.

- Types: Fats can be categorized into saturated, unsaturated (monounsaturated and polyunsaturated), and trans fats. Focus on consuming unsaturated fats, while limiting saturated fats and avoiding trans fats.
- Sources: Avocados, nuts (almonds, walnuts), seeds (chia, flax), olive oil, fatty fish (salmon, mackerel), and omega-3 supplements.

Micronutrients: Essential Vitamins and Minerals

While macronutrients provide the bulk of our energy needs, micronutrients—vitamins and minerals—play a crucial role in maintaining health, especially for endomorphic seniors. These essential nutrients support a wide range of bodily functions, from bone health to immune function, and are vital for preventing deficiencies and promoting overall well-being. In this sub-chapter, we will explore the importance of key vitamins and minerals, their sources, and practical tips for ensuring adequate intake.

Key Vitamins

1. Vitamin A

- Function: Supports vision, immune function, and skin health.
- Sources: Carrots, sweet potatoes, spinach, kale, and liver.
- Daily Requirement: Approximately 700-900 micrograms for seniors.
- Tips: Incorporate colorful fruits and vegetables into your diet to boost vitamin A intake.

2. Vitamin B Complex

- Function: Includes several vitamins (B1, B2, B3, B5, B6, B7, B9, B12) that collectively support energy production, red blood cell formation, and neurological function.
- Sources: Whole grains, eggs, dairy products, meat, legumes, and leafy greens.
- Daily Requirement: Varies by specific vitamin; for example, B12 is about 2.4 micrograms for seniors.
- Tips: Include a variety of B-vitamin-rich foods in your diet to ensure you get the full spectrum of benefits.

3. Vitamin C

- Function: Acts as an antioxidant, supports immune health, and aids in collagen production.
- Sources: Citrus fruits, strawberries, bell peppers, and broccoli.
- Daily Requirement: Approximately 75-90 milligrams for seniors.
- Tips: Snack on fresh fruits and vegetables to meet your vitamin C needs.

4. Vitamin D

- Function: Essential for calcium absorption, bone health, and immune function.
- Sources: Sunlight exposure, fatty fish (salmon, mackerel), fortified milk, and supplements.
- Daily Requirement: Approximately 800-1000 IU for seniors.
- Tips: Spend some time outdoors each day and consider a vitamin D supplement, especially in winter months or if you have limited sun exposure.

5. Vitamin E

- Function: Functions as an antioxidant, protecting cells from damage, and supports immune health.

- Sources: Nuts, seeds, spinach, and vegetable oils.
- Daily Requirement: Approximately 15 milligrams for seniors.
- Tips: Include nuts and seeds in your snacks and meals for a vitamin E boost.

6. Vitamin K

- Function: Important for blood clotting and bone health.
- Sources: Leafy greens (kale, spinach), broccoli, and Brussels sprouts.
- Daily Requirement: Approximately 90-120 micrograms for seniors.
- Tips: Add leafy greens to your salads and smoothies.

Key Minerals

1. Calcium

- Function: Vital for bone health, muscle function, and nerve signaling.
- Sources: Dairy products, fortified plant-based milks, leafy greens, and tofu.
- Daily Requirement: Approximately 1,200 milligrams for seniors.

- Tips: Consume dairy or fortified plant-based alternatives daily, and consider a calcium supplement if needed.

2. Magnesium

- Function: Supports muscle and nerve function, blood sugar control, and bone health.
- Sources: Nuts, seeds, whole grains, and leafy green vegetables.
- Daily Requirement: Approximately 320-420 milligrams for seniors.
- Tips: Include a variety of magnesium-rich foods in your diet to ensure adequate intake.

3. Iron

- Function: Essential for the production of hemoglobin, which carries oxygen in the blood.
- Sources: Red meat, poultry, fish, lentils, beans, and fortified cereals.
- Daily Requirement: Approximately 8 milligrams for seniors.
- Tips: Pair plant-based iron sources with vitamin C-rich foods to enhance absorption.

4. Zinc

- Function: Supports immune function, wound healing, and DNA synthesis.
- Sources: Meat, shellfish, dairy products, nuts, and legumes.
- Daily Requirement: Approximately 8-11 milligrams for seniors.
- Tips: Include a mix of animal and plant-based zinc sources in your diet.

5. Potassium

- Function: Helps regulate fluid balance, muscle contractions, and nerve signals.
- Sources: Bananas, oranges, potatoes, spinach, and beans.
- Daily Requirement: Approximately 2,600-3,400 milligrams for seniors.
- Tips: Incorporate potassium-rich fruits and vegetables into your meals and snacks.

Adjusting Caloric Intake for Age and Activity Level

As we age, our body's metabolism and caloric needs change. For endomorphic seniors, adjusting caloric intake is crucial to maintain a healthy weight, support daily activities, and prevent chronic conditions.

Basal Metabolic Rate (BMR) is the number of calories your body needs at rest to maintain essential physiological functions like breathing, circulation, and cell production.

Factors Affecting BMR: Age, gender, weight, and body composition influence BMR. As we age, BMR typically decreases due to a loss of muscle mass and changes in hormonal levels.

Total Daily Energy Expenditure (TDEE) is the total number of calories your body needs in a day, including all activities.

Components: TDEE includes BMR, physical activity, and the thermic effect of food (calories burned during digestion).

Activity Levels: Sedentary, lightly active, moderately active, very active, and extra active lifestyles influence TDEE. Seniors often fall into the sedentary or lightly active categories but may vary.

Calculating Caloric Needs

1. Determine BMR

Formulas: The Harris-Benedict Equation or Mifflin-St Jeor Equation can estimate BMR.

Harris-Benedict (revised):

- Men: BMR = 88.362 + (13.397 × weight in kg) + (4.799 × height in cm) - (5.677 × age in years)
- Women: BMR = 447.593 + (9.247 × weight in kg) + (3.098 × height in cm) - (4.330 × age in years)

Mifflin-St Jeor:

- Men: BMR = (10 × weight in kg) + (6.25 × height in cm) - (5 × age in years) + 5
- Women: BMR = (10 × weight in kg) + (6.25 × height in cm) - (5 × age in years) - 161

2. Calculate TDEE

Activity Multipliers:

- Sedentary (little to no exercise): BMR × 1.2
- Lightly active (light exercise/sports 1-3 days/week): BMR × 1.375
- Moderately active (moderate exercise/sports 3-5 days/week): BMR × 1.55
- Very active (hard exercise/sports 6-7 days a week): BMR × 1.725
- Extra active (very hard exercise/sports & physical job or 2x training): BMR × 1.9

Adjusting for Age

1. Caloric Reduction

- Gradual Decrease: Caloric needs decrease with age, typically by 100-200 calories per decade after the age of 50.
- Monitoring: Regularly monitor weight and adjust caloric intake to maintain a healthy weight.

2. Focus on Nutrient Density

- Nutrient-Rich Foods: Prioritize foods high in vitamins, minerals, fiber, and protein but lower in empty calories (sugary and processed foods).
- Balanced Meals: Ensure meals include a variety of food groups to meet nutrient needs without excessive calories.

Adjusting for Activity Level

1. Sedentary Seniors

Caloric Needs: Typically require fewer calories due to lower activity levels.

Strategies:

- Incorporate low-impact activities like walking or gentle yoga to boost metabolism.

- Focus on portion control and avoid high-calorie snacks.

2. Active Seniors

Caloric Needs: Higher due to increased physical activity.

Strategies:

- Include balanced meals with a good mix of carbohydrates, proteins, and fats to fuel activity.
- Ensure adequate hydration and consider small, frequent meals to sustain energy levels.

Chapter 3: Crafting the Perfect Meal Plan

Creating Balanced and Nutritious Meals

Creating balanced and nutritious meals is essential for maintaining health, managing weight, and supporting overall well-being, especially for seniors with an endomorphic body type.

Principles of Meal Balance

1. Macronutrient Balance

- Carbohydrates: Should make up 45-65% of total daily calories. Focus on complex carbs like whole grains, fruits, and vegetables.
- Proteins: Should account for 10-35% of total daily calories. Include lean protein sources such as poultry, fish, beans, and legumes.
- Fats: Should constitute 20-35% of total daily calories. Opt for healthy fats from sources like avocados, nuts, seeds, and olive oil.

2. Micronutrient Inclusion

- Vitamins and Minerals: Ensure your meals are rich in essential vitamins and minerals by incorporating a variety of colorful fruits and vegetables.

- Fiber: Aim for 25-30 grams of fiber daily to support digestive health and satiety. Sources include whole grains, fruits, vegetables, and legumes.

3. Hydration

- Water Intake: Drink at least 8 glasses (64 ounces) of water daily, adjusting based on activity level and climate. Hydrate with water, herbal teas, and water-rich foods.

Portion Control

1. Understanding Portion Sizes

- Serving Sizes: Familiarize yourself with standard serving sizes for different food groups to avoid overeating.
- Portion Guides: Use tools like measuring cups, food scales, and portion control plates to manage serving sizes.

2. Visual Portion Cues

- Hand Method: Use your hand as a guide—palm size for protein, fist size for carbs, cupped hand for vegetables, and thumb size for fats.

- Plate Method: Fill half your plate with vegetables, one-quarter with lean protein, and one-quarter with whole grains or starchy vegetables.

Practical Tips for Meal Planning and Preparation

1. Meal Planning

- Weekly Plan: Create a weekly meal plan to ensure balanced and nutritious meals. Include a variety of food groups and consider portion sizes.
- Grocery List: Make a grocery list based on your meal plan to avoid impulse buys and ensure you have all necessary ingredients.

2. Meal Preparation

- Batch Cooking: Prepare larger quantities of meals and portion them into individual servings for the week. This saves time and ensures you have healthy options readily available.
- Healthy Cooking Methods: Opt for cooking methods like grilling, baking, steaming, and sautéing with minimal oil to retain nutrients and reduce added fats.

3. Incorporating Variety

- Rotate Foods: Rotate different types of proteins, vegetables, and grains to keep meals interesting and nutritionally balanced.

- Seasonal Produce: Use seasonal fruits and vegetables to enjoy fresh, flavorful, and nutrient-rich foods.

28-Day Sample Meal Plan

Week 1	
Day 1	
Breakfast	Greek yogurt with honey, mixed berries, and a sprinkle of granola.
Snack	Apple slices with almond butter.
Lunch	Quinoa salad with black beans, corn, bell peppers, and avocado.
Snack	Carrot sticks with hummus.
Dinner	Grilled salmon with roasted Brussels sprouts and sweet potato wedges.
Day 2	
Breakfast	Oatmeal with banana slices, chia seeds, and a dash of cinnamon.

Snack	A handful of mixed nuts.
Lunch	Turkey and avocado wrap with whole grain tortilla, lettuce, and tomato.
Snack	A small bowl of mixed berries.
Dinner	Baked chicken breast with quinoa and steamed broccoli.
Day 3	
Breakfast	Scrambled eggs with spinach, tomatoes, and whole grain toast.
Snack	Greek yogurt with a few nuts.
Lunch	Lentil soup with a side of mixed green salad.
Snack	Orange slices.
Dinner	Stir-fried tofu with mixed vegetables and brown rice.
Day 4	
Breakfast	Smoothie made with spinach, banana, berries, and almond milk.
Snack	Celery sticks with peanut butter.
Lunch	Grilled chicken Caesar salad with light dressing.
Snack	Afternoon Snack: A small handful of trail mix.
Dinner	Baked cod with quinoa and roasted asparagus.
Day 5	

Breakfast	Whole grain waffles with fresh berries and a drizzle of maple syrup.
Snack	Greek yogurt with a few sunflower seeds.
Lunch	Chickpea salad with cucumbers, tomatoes, and feta cheese.
Snack	Sliced bell peppers with hummus.
Dinner	Turkey meatballs with spaghetti squash and marinara sauce.

Day 6

Breakfast	Smoothie bowl topped with granola, sliced banana, and berries.
Snack	Cottage cheese with pineapple chunks.
Lunch	Tuna salad sandwich on whole grain bread with a side of mixed greens.
Snack	A small handful of almonds.
Dinner	Grilled shrimp with brown rice and sautéed spinach.

Day 7

Breakfast	Scrambled eggs with smoked salmon and whole grain toast.
Snack	Fresh fruit salad.
Lunch	Vegetable stir-fry with tofu and quinoa.
Snack	A small bowl of mixed nuts.

| Dinner | Baked chicken thighs with roasted carrots and parsnips. |

Week 2

Day 8

Breakfast	Overnight oats with almond milk, chia seeds, and blueberries.
Snack	A pear with a few walnuts.
Lunch	Greek salad with grilled chicken.
Snack	A few slices of cucumber with tzatziki sauce.
Dinner	Baked tilapia with wild rice and steamed green beans.

Day 9

Breakfast	Smoothie made with kale, pineapple, mango, and coconut water.
Snack	Cottage cheese with a few berries.
Lunch	Turkey and avocado wrap with whole grain tortilla.
Snack	Afternoon Snack: Baby carrots with hummus.
Dinner	Grilled steak with roasted sweet potatoes and Brussels sprouts.

Day 10

Breakfast	Greek yogurt with honey, mixed nuts, and seeds.
Snack	An apple with almond butter.

Lunch	Lunch: Quinoa and black bean salad with corn, bell peppers, and cilantro.
Snack	A small handful of trail mix.
Dinner	Baked chicken breast with quinoa and steamed broccoli.
Day 11	
Breakfast	Scrambled eggs with spinach, tomatoes, and whole grain toast.
Snack	Fresh fruit salad.
Lunch	Lentil soup with a side of mixed green salad.
Snack	Celery sticks with peanut butter.
Dinner	Stir-fried tofu with mixed vegetables and brown rice.
Day 12	
Breakfast	Smoothie made with spinach, banana, berries, and almond milk.
Snack	Cottage cheese with pineapple chunks.
Lunch	Grilled chicken Caesar salad with light dressing.
Snack	A small handful of almonds.
Dinner	Baked cod with quinoa and roasted asparagus.
Day 13	

Breakfast	Whole grain waffles with fresh berries and a drizzle of maple syrup.
Snack	Greek yogurt with a few sunflower seeds.
Lunch	Chickpea salad with cucumbers, tomatoes, and feta cheese.
Snack	Sliced bell peppers with hummus.
Dinner	Turkey meatballs with spaghetti squash and marinara sauce.
Day 14	
Breakfast	Smoothie bowl topped with granola, sliced banana, and berries.
Snack	Cottage cheese with pineapple chunks.
Lunch	Tuna salad sandwich on whole grain bread with a side of mixed greens.
Snack	A small handful of almonds.
Dinner	Grilled shrimp with brown rice and sautéed spinach.
Week 3	
Day 15	
Breakfast	Greek yogurt with honey, mixed berries, and a sprinkle of granola.
Snack	Apple slices with almond butter.
Lunch	Quinoa salad with black beans, corn, bell peppers, and avocado.

Snack	Carrot sticks with hummus.
Dinner	Grilled salmon with roasted Brussels sprouts and sweet potato wedges.

Day 16

Breakfast	Oatmeal with banana slices, chia seeds, and a dash of cinnamon.
Snack	A handful of mixed nuts.
Lunch	Turkey and avocado wrap with whole grain tortilla, lettuce, and tomato.
Snack	A small bowl of mixed berries.
Dinner	Baked chicken breast with quinoa and steamed broccoli.

Day 17

Breakfast	Scrambled eggs with spinach, tomatoes, and whole grain toast.
Snack	Greek yogurt with a few nuts.
Lunch	Lentil soup with a side of mixed green salad.
Snack	Orange slices.
Dinner	Stir-fried tofu with mixed vegetables and brown rice.

Day 18

Breakfast	Smoothie made with spinach, banana, berries, and almond milk.
Snack	Celery sticks with peanut butter.

Lunch	Grilled chicken Caesar salad with light dressing.
Snack	A small handful of trail mix.
Dinner	Baked cod with quinoa and roasted asparagus.

Day 19

Breakfast	Whole grain waffles with fresh berries and a drizzle of maple syrup.
Snack	Greek yogurt with a few sunflower seeds.
Lunch	Chickpea salad with cucumbers, tomatoes, and feta cheese.
Snack	Sliced bell peppers with hummus.
Dinner	Turkey meatballs with spaghetti squash and marinara sauce.

Day 20

Breakfast	Smoothie bowl topped with granola, sliced banana, and berries.
Snack	Cottage cheese with pineapple chunks.
Lunch	Tuna salad sandwich on whole grain bread with a side of mixed greens.
Snack	A small handful of almonds.
Dinner	Grilled shrimp with brown rice and sautéed spinach.

Day 21

Breakfast	Scrambled eggs with smoked salmon and whole grain toast.
Snack	Fresh fruit salad.
Lunch	Vegetable stir-fry with tofu and quinoa.
Snack	A small bowl of mixed nuts.
Dinner	Baked chicken thighs with roasted carrots and parsnips.

Week 4

Day 22

Breakfast	Overnight oats with almond milk, chia seeds, and blueberries.
Snack	A pear with a few walnuts.
Lunch	Greek salad with grilled chicken.
Snack	A few slices of cucumber with tzatziki sauce.
Dinner	Baked tilapia with wild rice and steamed green beans.

Day 23

Breakfast	Smoothie made with kale, pineapple, mango, and coconut water.
Snack	Cottage cheese with a few berries.
Lunch	Turkey and avocado wrap with whole grain tortilla.
Snack	Baby carrots with hummus.

Dinner	Grilled steak with roasted sweet potatoes and Brussels sprouts.
Day 24	
Breakfast	Greek yogurt with honey, mixed nuts, and seeds.
Snack	An apple with almond butter.
Lunch	Quinoa and black bean salad with corn, bell peppers, and cilantro.
Snack	A small handful of trail mix.
Dinner	Baked chicken breast with quinoa and steamed broccoli.
Day 25	
Breakfast	Scrambled eggs with spinach, tomatoes, and whole grain toast.
Snack	Fresh fruit salad.
Lunch	Lentil soup with a side of mixed green salad.
Snack	Celery sticks with peanut butter.
Dinner	Stir-fried tofu with mixed vegetables and brown rice.
Day 26	
Breakfast	Smoothie made with spinach, banana, berries, and almond milk.
Snack	Cottage cheese with pineapple chunks.

Lunch	Grilled chicken Caesar salad with light dressing.
Snack	A small handful of almonds.
Dinner	Baked cod with quinoa and roasted asparagus.

Day 27

Breakfast	Whole grain waffles with fresh berries and a drizzle of maple syrup.
Snack	Greek yogurt with a few sunflower seeds.
Lunch	Chickpea salad with cucumbers, tomatoes, and feta cheese.
Snack	Sliced bell peppers with hummus.
Dinner	Turkey meatballs with spaghetti squash and marinara sauce.

Day 28

Breakfast	Smoothie bowl topped with granola, sliced banana, and berries.
Snack	Cottage cheese with pineapple chunks.
Lunch	Tuna salad sandwich on whole grain bread with a side of mixed greens.
Snack	A small handful of almonds.
Dinner	Grilled shrimp with brown rice and sautéed spinach.

Shopping Lists

Produce	
Bananas	Apples
Carrots	Celery
Bell peppers	Avocado
Tomatoes	Spinach
Kale	Broccoli
Sweet potatoes	Brussels sprouts
Asparagus	Cucumbers
Pears	Mango
Oranges	Pineapple
Mixed greens (lettuce, arugula)	
Mixed berries (blueberries, strawberries, raspberries)	

Proteins	
Greek yogurt	Almond butter
Chicken breasts	Salmon
Tofu	Black beans
Turkey breast	Eggs
Cod	

Grains and Legumes	
Quinoa	Whole grain bread
Whole grain tortillas	Granola

Oatmeal	Brown rice
Spaghetti squash	

Dairy and Alternatives	
Almond milk	Cottage cheese
Feta cheese	

Snacks and Extras	
Mixed nuts	Sunflower seeds
Hummus	Trail mix

Condiments and Spices	
Olive oil	Balsamic vinegar
Chia seeds	Honey
Cinnamon	Tzatziki sauce

Pantry Essentials

Grains and Legumes	
Brown rice	Quinoa
Whole grain pasta	Lentils
Black beans	Chickpeas

Oils and Vinegars	
Extra virgin olive oil	Coconut oil
Balsamic vinegar	Apple cider vinegar

Nuts and Seeds	
Almonds	Walnuts

| Chia seeds | Flaxseeds |
| Pumpkin seeds | Sunflower seeds |

Herbs and Spices

Cinnamon	Turmeric
Cumin	Paprika
Oregano	Basil
Thyme	Bay leaves
Rosemary	Black pepper
Sea salt	

Canned Goods

| Canned tomatoes | Tomato paste |
| Coconut milk | Low-sodium vegetable broth |

Baking Essentials

| Whole wheat flour | Almond flour |
| Baking powder | Baking soda |

Condiments and Sauces

Low-sodium soy sauce	Dijon mustard
Honey	Maple syrup
Tzatziki sauce	Hot sauce

Other Essentials

Rolled oats	Whole grain bread
Whole grain tortillas	Granola
Greek yogurt	Almond milk

Chapter 4: Recipes for Endomorph Seniors

Greek Yogurt Parfait with Berries and Nuts	
Ingredients	Greek yogurt, mixed berries (blueberries, strawberries, raspberries), almonds, chia seeds, honey.
Instructions	Layer Greek yogurt with mixed berries. Top with almonds, chia seeds, and a drizzle of honey.

Veggie Omelette	
Ingredients	Eggs, spinach, bell peppers, tomatoes, onions, feta cheese, olive oil.
Instructions	Sauté vegetables in olive oil, then add beaten eggs. Cook until set and sprinkle with feta cheese.

Overnight Chia Pudding	
Ingredients	Chia seeds, almond milk, vanilla extract, honey, fresh fruit (such as mango or kiwi).
Instructions	Mix chia seeds with almond milk, vanilla extract, and honey. Refrigerate overnight. Serve with fresh fruit.

Avocado Toast with Poached Egg

Ingredients	Whole grain bread, avocado, eggs, lemon juice, salt, pepper, red pepper flakes.
Instructions	Mash avocado with lemon juice, salt, and pepper. Spread on toasted bread and top with a poached egg and red pepper flakes.

Quinoa Breakfast Bowl

Ingredients	Cooked quinoa, almond milk, sliced almonds, blueberries, cinnamon, honey.
Instructions	Warm cooked quinoa with almond milk. Top with sliced almonds, blueberries, cinnamon, and a drizzle of honey.

Smoothie Bowl

Ingredients	Frozen berries, banana, spinach, almond milk, chia seeds, granola.
Instructions	Blend frozen berries, banana, spinach, and almond milk until smooth. Pour into a bowl and top with chia seeds and granola.

Oatmeal with Flaxseeds and Fruit

Ingredients	Rolled oats, water or almond milk, ground flaxseeds, apple slices, cinnamon, walnuts.
Instructions	Cook oats with water or almond milk. Stir in ground flaxseeds and top with apple slices, cinnamon, and walnuts.

Cottage Cheese and Fruit

Ingredients	Cottage cheese, pineapple chunks, sunflower seeds, honey.
Instructions	Serve cottage cheese with pineapple chunks, sunflower seeds, and a drizzle of honey.

Sweet Potato Hash with Eggs

Ingredients	Sweet potatoes, bell peppers, onions, eggs, olive oil, salt, pepper.
Instructions	Sauté diced sweet potatoes, bell peppers, and onions in olive oil. Cook until tender. Serve with fried or poached eggs on top.

Almond Butter and Banana Sandwich

Ingredients	Whole grain bread, almond butter, banana, cinnamon.
Instructions	Spread almond butter on whole grain bread. Top with banana slices and a sprinkle of cinnamon.

Breakfast Burrito

Ingredients	Whole grain tortilla, scrambled eggs, black beans, spinach, salsa, avocado.
Instructions	Fill a whole grain tortilla with scrambled eggs, black beans, spinach, salsa, and avocado slices. Roll up and enjoy.

Protein Pancakes

Ingredients	Oats, banana, eggs, vanilla extract, baking powder, cinnamon, fresh berries.
Instructions	Blend oats, banana, eggs, vanilla extract, baking powder, and cinnamon to form a batter. Cook pancakes on a non-stick skillet. Serve with fresh berries.

Spinach and Feta Breakfast Wrap

Ingredients	Whole grain wrap, scrambled eggs, spinach, feta cheese, cherry tomatoes.
Instructions	Fill a whole grain wrap with scrambled eggs, spinach, feta cheese, and cherry tomatoes. Wrap and serve.

Apple Cinnamon Overnight Oats

Ingredients	Rolled oats, almond milk, grated apple, cinnamon, walnuts, honey.
Instructions	Mix rolled oats, almond milk, grated apple, cinnamon, and honey. Refrigerate overnight. Top with walnuts before serving.

Tofu Scramble

Ingredients	Tofu, turmeric, spinach, bell peppers, onions, nutritional yeast, olive oil.
Instructions	Crumble tofu and sauté with turmeric, spinach, bell peppers, onions, and olive oil.

| | Sprinkle with nutritional yeast for a cheesy flavor. |

Grilled Chicken and Quinoa Salad

Ingredients	Grilled chicken breast, quinoa, mixed greens, cherry tomatoes, cucumbers, red onion, olive oil, lemon juice, salt, pepper.
Instructions	Toss grilled chicken and quinoa with mixed greens, cherry tomatoes, cucumbers, and red onion. Drizzle with olive oil and lemon juice, and season with salt and pepper.

Lentil Soup

Ingredients	Lentils, carrots, celery, onions, garlic, vegetable broth, tomatoes, spinach, cumin, paprika, olive oil.
Instructions	Sauté onions, carrots, celery, and garlic in olive oil. Add lentils, vegetable broth, tomatoes, spinach, and spices. Simmer until lentils are tender.

Turkey and Avocado Wrap

Ingredients	Whole grain wrap, sliced turkey breast, avocado, lettuce, tomato, mustard.

Instructions	Layer sliced turkey, avocado, lettuce, and tomato on a whole grain wrap. Spread mustard and roll up.

Greek Salad with Grilled Shrimp

Ingredients	Grilled shrimp, mixed greens, cucumbers, cherry tomatoes, Kalamata olives, red onion, feta cheese, olive oil, lemon juice, oregano.
Instructions	Combine grilled shrimp with mixed greens, cucumbers, cherry tomatoes, olives, and red onion. Top with feta cheese and drizzle with olive oil and lemon juice. Sprinkle with oregano.

Chickpea and Spinach Stew

Ingredients	Chickpeas, spinach, onions, garlic, tomatoes, vegetable broth, cumin, paprika, olive oil.
Instructions	Sauté onions and garlic in olive oil. Add chickpeas, tomatoes, vegetable broth, and spices. Simmer until flavors meld. Stir in spinach until wilted.

Tuna Salad Lettuce Wraps

Ingredients	Tuna, Greek yogurt, celery, red onion, dill, lemon juice, Romaine lettuce leaves.

Instructions	Mix tuna with Greek yogurt, chopped celery, red onion, dill, and lemon juice. Serve in Romaine lettuce leaves.

Stuffed Bell Peppers

Ingredients	Bell peppers, ground turkey, quinoa, black beans, corn, tomatoes, onions, cumin, chili powder, cheese (optional).
Instructions	Hollow out bell peppers and fill with a mixture of cooked ground turkey, quinoa, black beans, corn, tomatoes, onions, and spices. Top with cheese if desired and bake until peppers are tender.

Eggplant and Chickpea Curry

Ingredients	Eggplant, chickpeas, onions, garlic, tomatoes, coconut milk, curry powder, cumin, coriander, olive oil.
Instructions	Sauté onions and garlic in olive oil. Add eggplant and cook until tender. Stir in chickpeas, tomatoes, coconut milk, and spices. Simmer until flavors combine.

Spinach and Feta Stuffed Chicken

Ingredients	Chicken breasts, spinach, feta cheese, garlic, olive oil, lemon juice.

| Instructions | Sauté spinach and garlic in olive oil. Mix with feta cheese and stuff into chicken breasts. Bake until chicken is cooked through and serve with a side salad. |

Salmon and Asparagus

Ingredients	Salmon fillets, asparagus, olive oil, lemon zest, salt, pepper.
Instructions	Roast salmon fillets and asparagus with olive oil, lemon zest, salt, and pepper until salmon is flaky and asparagus is tender.

Cauliflower Rice Stir-Fry

Ingredients	Cauliflower rice, mixed vegetables (carrots, bell peppers, peas), tofu, soy sauce, garlic, ginger, olive oil.
Instructions	Sauté mixed vegetables and tofu in olive oil with garlic and ginger. Add cauliflower rice and soy sauce. Cook until heated through.

Zucchini Noodles with Pesto

Ingredients	Zucchini noodles, pesto (basil, pine nuts, garlic, Parmesan, olive oil), cherry tomatoes.

Instructions	Toss zucchini noodles with pesto and cherry tomatoes. Serve raw or lightly sautéed.

Beef and Broccoli

Ingredients	Lean beef strips, broccoli florets, soy sauce, garlic, ginger, olive oil.
Instructions	Sauté beef strips in olive oil with garlic and ginger. Add broccoli and soy sauce, and cook until broccoli is tender.

Hummus and Veggie Plate

Ingredients	Hummus, carrot sticks, cucumber slices, bell pepper strips, cherry tomatoes, whole grain pita bread.
Instructions	Serve hummus with an assortment of fresh vegetables and whole grain pita bread.

Turkey Chili

Ingredients	Ground turkey, kidney beans, black beans, tomatoes, onions, garlic, chili powder, cumin, olive oil.
Instructions	Sauté onions and garlic in olive oil. Add ground turkey and cook until browned. Stir in beans, tomatoes, and spices. Simmer until flavors meld.

Baked Salmon with Roasted Vegetables

Ingredients	Salmon fillets, broccoli, carrots, bell peppers, olive oil, lemon zest, salt, pepper.
Instructions	Season salmon with lemon zest, salt, and pepper. Roast salmon and vegetables in olive oil until salmon is flaky and vegetables are tender.

Turkey and Spinach Stuffed Peppers

Ingredients	Bell peppers, ground turkey, spinach, quinoa, garlic, onions, tomato sauce, Italian seasoning.
Instructions	Cook ground turkey with garlic, onions, and spinach. Mix with cooked quinoa and tomato sauce. Stuff into bell peppers and bake until peppers are tender.

Lentil and Vegetable Stew

Ingredients	Lentils, carrots, celery, tomatoes, spinach, onions, garlic, vegetable broth, thyme, cumin.
Instructions	Sauté onions and garlic, then add lentils, vegetables, broth, and spices. Simmer until lentils and vegetables are tender.

Grilled Chicken with Quinoa and Asparagus

Ingredients	Grilled chicken breast, quinoa, asparagus, lemon juice, olive oil, salt, pepper.
Instructions	Grill chicken breast and serve with cooked quinoa and steamed asparagus, drizzled with olive oil and lemon juice.

Shrimp and Avocado Salad

Ingredients	Cooked shrimp, mixed greens, avocado, cherry tomatoes, cucumbers, red onion, olive oil, lime juice.
Instructions	Toss shrimp and vegetables with olive oil and lime juice. Serve chilled.

Eggplant Parmesan

Ingredients	Eggplant slices, marinara sauce, mozzarella cheese, Parmesan cheese, basil, whole grain breadcrumbs.
Instructions	Bread and bake eggplant slices, then layer with marinara sauce and cheese. Bake until cheese is melted and bubbly.

Tofu and Vegetable Stir-Fry

Ingredients	Firm tofu, bell peppers, broccoli, snow peas, soy sauce, ginger, garlic, olive oil.
Instructions	Sauté tofu and vegetables in olive oil with ginger and garlic. Add soy sauce and cook until vegetables are tender.

Beef and Vegetable Kebabs

Ingredients	Lean beef cubes, bell peppers, onions, cherry tomatoes, zucchini, olive oil, garlic, rosemary.
Instructions	Thread beef and vegetables onto skewers. Brush with olive oil and garlic, and grill until beef is cooked to your liking.

Chickpea and Spinach Curry

Ingredients	Chickpeas, spinach, onions, garlic, tomatoes, coconut milk, curry powder, cumin.
Instructions	Sauté onions and garlic, add chickpeas, tomatoes, coconut milk, and spices. Simmer until flavors meld and stir in spinach until wilted.

Baked Cod with Lemon and Dill

Ingredients	Cod fillets, lemon slices, fresh dill, olive oil, salt, pepper.
Instructions	Place cod fillets on a baking sheet, top with lemon slices and dill, drizzle with olive oil, and bake until fish is flaky.

Chicken and Vegetable Skillet

Ingredients	Chicken thighs, zucchini, bell peppers, cherry tomatoes, garlic, olive oil, Italian seasoning.
Instructions	Sauté chicken thighs until browned, then add vegetables and cook until chicken is fully cooked and vegetables are tender.

Cauliflower Rice with Grilled Shrimp

Ingredients	Grilled shrimp, cauliflower rice, garlic, olive oil, parsley, lemon juice.
Instructions	Sauté cauliflower rice with garlic in olive oil, then top with grilled shrimp and a squeeze of lemon juice.

Turkey Meatballs with Zucchini Noodles

Ingredients	Ground turkey, egg, whole grain breadcrumbs, garlic, marinara sauce, zucchini noodles.
Instructions	Mix ground turkey with egg, breadcrumbs, and garlic. Form meatballs and bake. Serve with zucchini noodles and marinara sauce.

Stuffed Acorn Squash

Ingredients	Acorn squash, quinoa, dried cranberries, pecans, spinach, olive oil, maple syrup.
Instructions	Roast halved acorn squash, then stuff with a mixture of cooked quinoa, dried

	cranberries, pecans, spinach, olive oil, and maple syrup.

Black Bean and Sweet Potato Tacos

Ingredients	Black beans, sweet potatoes, whole grain tortillas, avocado, salsa, cilantro, cumin, chili powder.
Instructions	Roast sweet potatoes with cumin and chili powder. Serve in tortillas with black beans, avocado, salsa, and cilantro.

Healthy Snacks and Desserts

Snacks

Greek Yogurt with Berries

Ingredients	Greek yogurt, mixed berries (blueberries, strawberries, raspberries), honey (optional).
Instructions	Top Greek yogurt with a handful of mixed berries. Drizzle with honey if desired.

Veggie Sticks with Hummus

Ingredients	Carrot sticks, celery sticks, bell pepper strips, hummus.
Instructions	Serve a variety of fresh vegetable sticks with a side of hummus for dipping.

Apple Slices with Almond Butter

Ingredients	Apple slices, almond butter, cinnamon.
Instructions	Spread almond butter on apple slices and sprinkle with a pinch of cinnamon.

Hard-Boiled Eggs

Ingredients	Eggs, salt, pepper.
Instructions	Boil eggs, peel, and season with a little salt and pepper.

Cottage Cheese with Pineapple

Ingredients	Cottage cheese, pineapple chunks.
Instructions	Mix cottage cheese with fresh pineapple chunks.

Avocado Toast

Ingredients	Whole grain bread, avocado, lemon juice, salt, pepper, red pepper flakes.
Instructions	Mash avocado with lemon juice, salt, and pepper. Spread on toasted whole grain bread and sprinkle with red pepper flakes.

Mixed Nuts and Seeds

Ingredients	Almonds, walnuts, sunflower seeds, pumpkin seeds.
Instructions	Combine a mix of nuts and seeds for a satisfying and nutrient-dense snack.

Edamame

Ingredients	Edamame, sea salt.
Instructions	Steam edamame and sprinkle with sea salt.

Rice Cakes with Nut Butter

Ingredients	Rice cakes, almond butter or peanut butter, banana slices.
Instructions	Spread nut butter on rice cakes and top with banana slices.

Chia Seed Pudding

Ingredients	Chia seeds, almond milk, vanilla extract, honey.
Instructions	Mix chia seeds with almond milk, vanilla extract, and a touch of honey. Refrigerate until it thickens.

Desserts

Dark Chocolate and Almonds

Ingredients	Dark chocolate (70% or higher), almonds.
Instructions	Pair a few squares of dark chocolate with a handful of almonds.

Baked Apple with Cinnamon

Ingredients	Apple, cinnamon, walnuts, honey.
Instructions	Core an apple and fill it with chopped walnuts and a sprinkle of cinnamon. Drizzle with honey and bake until tender.

Frozen Yogurt Bark

Ingredients	Greek yogurt, mixed berries, honey, chopped nuts.
Instructions	Spread Greek yogurt on a baking sheet, top with berries, honey, and chopped nuts. Freeze until firm, then break into pieces.

Fruit Salad

Ingredients	A mix of favorite fruits (such as strawberries, kiwi, mango, blueberries), mint leaves, lime juice.
Instructions	Toss mixed fruits with a few mint leaves and a squeeze of lime juice.

Banana Ice Cream

Ingredients	Frozen bananas, a splash of almond milk, vanilla extract.
Instructions	Blend frozen bananas with almond milk and vanilla extract until smooth and creamy.

Special Diet Considerations Options

Gluten-Free Options

Quinoa and Vegetable Stir-Fry

Ingredients	Quinoa, bell peppers, broccoli, snap peas, carrots, gluten-free soy sauce, garlic, olive oil.

| Instructions | Cook quinoa and set aside. Sauté vegetables in olive oil with garlic, add quinoa and gluten-free soy sauce, and stir-fry until heated through. |

Grilled Chicken with Sweet Potato and Kale

Ingredients	Chicken breast, sweet potatoes, kale, olive oil, garlic, lemon juice.
Instructions	Grill chicken breast and serve with roasted sweet potatoes and sautéed kale with garlic and lemon juice.

Lentil and Spinach Soup

Ingredients	Lentils, spinach, carrots, celery, onions, garlic, vegetable broth, olive oil.
Instructions	Sauté onions, carrots, celery, and garlic in olive oil. Add lentils and vegetable broth, simmer until lentils are tender, and stir in spinach.

Stuffed Bell Peppers

Ingredients	Bell peppers, ground turkey, quinoa, tomatoes, onions, garlic, Italian seasoning.
Instructions	Cook ground turkey with onions, garlic, and Italian seasoning. Mix with cooked quinoa and tomatoes. Stuff into bell peppers and bake.

Salmon with Asparagus

Ingredients	Salmon fillets, asparagus, olive oil, lemon, garlic, salt, pepper.
Instructions	Roast salmon fillets and asparagus with olive oil, garlic, lemon, salt, and pepper until cooked through.

Dairy-Free Options

Chicken and Avocado Salad

Ingredients	Grilled chicken breast, mixed greens, avocado, cherry tomatoes, cucumbers, olive oil, lemon juice.
Instructions	Mix grilled chicken with greens, avocado, cherry tomatoes, and cucumbers. Dress with olive oil and lemon juice.

Turkey and Vegetable Lettuce Wraps

Ingredients	Ground turkey, bell peppers, onions, garlic, lettuce leaves, soy sauce.
Instructions	Sauté ground turkey with bell peppers, onions, and garlic. Serve in lettuce leaves with a drizzle of soy sauce.

Baked Cod with Vegetable Medley

Ingredients	Cod fillets, mixed vegetables (zucchini, bell peppers, cherry tomatoes), olive oil, lemon, herbs.

| Instructions | Bake cod and vegetables with olive oil, lemon, and herbs until fish is flaky and vegetables are tender. |

Tofu and Vegetable Stir-Fry

| Ingredients | Firm tofu, broccoli, bell peppers, snap peas, gluten-free soy sauce, garlic, ginger, olive oil. |
| Instructions | Sauté tofu and vegetables in olive oil with garlic and ginger. Add gluten-free soy sauce and stir-fry until heated through. |

Coconut Curry Chicken

| Ingredients | Chicken breast, coconut milk, curry powder, onions, garlic, bell peppers, spinach. |
| Instructions | Sauté onions and garlic, add chicken and curry powder, then stir in coconut milk and bell peppers. Simmer until chicken is cooked, then add spinach until wilted. |

Low-Sodium Options

Herb-Roasted Chicken and Vegetables

| Ingredients | Chicken breast, carrots, Brussels sprouts, olive oil, garlic, rosemary, thyme. |

Instructions	Roast chicken and vegetables with olive oil, garlic, rosemary, and thyme until cooked through.

Lemon Garlic Shrimp and Zoodles

Ingredients	Shrimp, zucchini noodles, olive oil, garlic, lemon, parsley.
Instructions	Sauté shrimp in olive oil with garlic and lemon juice. Serve over zucchini noodles and garnish with parsley.

Beef and Vegetable Kebabs

Ingredients	Lean beef cubes, bell peppers, onions, cherry tomatoes, zucchini, olive oil, garlic, rosemary.
Instructions	Thread beef and vegetables onto skewers, brush with olive oil and garlic, and grill until beef is cooked to your liking.

Spinach and Mushroom Omelette

Ingredients	Eggs, spinach, mushrooms, onions, olive oil, black pepper.
Instructions	Sauté mushrooms and onions in olive oil. Add spinach until wilted, then pour in beaten eggs. Cook until omelette is set.

Baked Sweet Potato with Black Beans and Avocado

Ingredients	Sweet potatoes, black beans, avocado, cherry tomatoes, cilantro, lime juice.
Instructions	Bake sweet potatoes until tender. Top with black beans, diced avocado, cherry tomatoes, cilantro, and a squeeze of lime juice.

Chapter 5: Exercise Essentials for Endomorph Seniors

Understanding Endomorph Fitness Needs

For seniors with an endomorphic body type, fitness goals often revolve around maintaining a healthy weight, improving cardiovascular health, increasing muscle mass, and enhancing overall mobility and flexibility. Specific goals may include:

- Weight management: Reducing body fat while maintaining or increasing lean muscle mass.
- Cardiovascular health: Improving heart and lung function to reduce the risk of chronic diseases.
- Muscle strength: Building and preserving muscle mass to support daily activities and prevent age-related muscle loss.
- Flexibility and mobility: Enhancing joint flexibility and overall mobility to maintain independence and reduce the risk of falls.

Exercise Selection for Endomorphs

Endomorphs benefit from a combination of cardiovascular exercise, strength training, and flexibility exercises. Each type of exercise plays a vital role in achieving the fitness goals mentioned above.

1. Cardiovascular Exercise

Cardiovascular exercise is essential for burning calories, improving heart health, and increasing metabolism.

2. Strength Training

Strength training is crucial for building and preserving muscle mass, boosting metabolism, and supporting bone health

3. Flexibility and Mobility Exercises

Flexibility and mobility exercises help improve the range of motion, reduce stiffness, and enhance overall movement.

Beginner Workout Plan

Day 1: Cardio and Flexibility
Warm-Up (5-10 minutes) • Light walking or marching in place • Gentle arm circles and shoulder rolls
Cardio (20 minutes) • Brisk walking or low-impact aerobics

Flexibility (10 minutes)

- Neck stretches: Hold for 15-30 seconds each side
- Shoulder stretches: Hold for 15-30 seconds each side
- Hamstring stretches: Hold for 15-30 seconds each leg
- Calf stretches: Hold for 15-30 seconds each leg

Cool-Down (5 minutes)

- Slow walking and deep breathing

Day 2: Strength Training and Balance

Warm-Up (5-10 minutes)

- Light walking or gentle stretching

Strength Training (20 minutes)

- Chair squats: 2 sets of 10-12 repetitions
- Wall push-ups: 2 sets of 10-12 repetitions
- Seated bicep curls (using light weights or resistance bands): 2 sets of 10-12 repetitions
- Seated leg lifts: 2 sets of 10-12 repetitions

Balance (10 minutes)

- Heel-to-toe walking: 2 sets of 10 steps
- Standing on one leg: 2 sets of 15-30 seconds each leg

Cool-Down (5 minutes)

- Gentle stretching and deep breathing

Day 3: Cardio and Mobility

Warm-Up (5-10 minutes)

- Light walking or marching in place

Cardio (20 minutes)

- Cycling on a stationary bike or dancing

Mobility (10 minutes)

- Cat-cow stretch: 1-2 minutes

- Hip flexor stretch: Hold for 15-30 seconds each side

- Ankle circles: 1-2 minutes

Cool-Down (5 minutes)

- Slow walking and deep breathing

Day 4: Rest or Active Recovery

Active Recovery (Optional)

- Gentle yoga or stretching for 20-30 minutes

- Leisurely walking for 15-20 minutes

Relaxation

- Deep breathing exercises or meditation for 5-10 minutes

Day 5: Strength Training and Flexibility

Warm-Up (5-10 minutes)

- Light walking or gentle stretching

Strength Training (20 minutes)

- Seated leg presses (using resistance bands or no weights): 2 sets of 10-12 repetitions
- Overhead shoulder presses (using light weights or resistance bands): 2 sets of 10-12 repetitions
- Seated rows (using resistance bands): 2 sets of 10-12 repetitions
- Standing calf raises: 2 sets of 10-12 repetitions

Flexibility (10 minutes)

- Chest stretch: Hold for 15-30 seconds
- Quadriceps stretch: Hold for 15-30 seconds each leg
- Side stretches: Hold for 15-30 seconds each side

Cool-Down (5 minutes)

- Gentle stretching and deep breathing

Day 6: Cardio and Balance

Warm-Up (5-10 minutes)

- Light walking or marching in place

Cardio (20 minutes)

- Swimming or water aerobics (if accessible)

Balance (10 minutes)

- Balance board exercises: 2 sets of 10-12 repetitions

- Stability ball exercises (seated or standing): 2 sets of 10-12 repetitions

Cool-Down (5 minutes)

- Slow walking and deep breathing

Day 7: Rest or Active Recovery

Active Recovery (Optional)

- Gentle yoga or stretching for 20-30 minutes
- Leisurely walking for 15-20 minutes

Relaxation

- Deep breathing exercises or meditation for 5-10 minutes

Intermediate Workout Plan

Day 1: Cardio and Flexibility

Warm-Up (5-10 minutes)

- Light jogging or brisk walking
- Dynamic stretches: leg swings, arm circles, and torso twists

Cardio (30 minutes)

- Power walking, light jogging, or low-impact aerobics

Flexibility (10 minutes)

- Neck stretches: Hold for 15-30 seconds each side

- Shoulder stretches: Hold for 15-30 seconds each side

- Hamstring stretches: Hold for 15-30 seconds each leg

- Calf stretches: Hold for 15-30 seconds each leg

Cool-Down (5 minutes)

- Slow walking and deep breathing

Day 2: Strength Training and Balance

Warm-Up (5-10 minutes)

- Light jogging or gentle stretching

Strength Training (30 minutes)

- Squats: 3 sets of 12-15 repetitions

- Push-ups (modified or standard): 3 sets of 12-15 repetitions

- Dumbbell rows: 3 sets of 12-15 repetitions each side

- Lunges: 3 sets of 12-15 repetitions each leg

- Bicep curls: 3 sets of 12-15 repetitions

- Tricep extensions: 3 sets of 12-15 repetitions

Balance (10 minutes)

- Heel-to-toe walking: 2 sets of 15 steps

- Single-leg stands: 3 sets of 20-30 seconds each leg

Cool-Down (5 minutes)

* Gentle stretching and deep breathing

Day 3: Cardio and Mobility

Warm-Up (5-10 minutes)

* Light jogging or marching in place

Cardio (30 minutes)

* Cycling on a stationary bike or dancing

Mobility (10 minutes)

* Cat-cow stretch: 1-2 minutes
* Hip flexor stretch: Hold for 15-30 seconds each side
* Ankle circles: 1-2 minutes

Cool-Down (5 minutes)

* Slow walking and deep breathing

Day 4: Active Recovery

Active Recovery (30-40 minutes)

* Gentle yoga or stretching
* Leisurely walking or swimming

Relaxation

* Deep breathing exercises or meditation for 10-15 minutes

Day 5: Strength Training and Flexibility

Warm-Up (5-10 minutes)

- Light jogging or gentle stretching

Strength Training (30 minutes)

- Deadlifts (using light weights or resistance bands): 3 sets of 12-15 repetitions
- Overhead shoulder presses: 3 sets of 12-15 repetitions
- Seated rows: 3 sets of 12-15 repetitions
- Step-ups: 3 sets of 12-15 repetitions each leg
- Seated leg presses: 3 sets of 12-15 repetitions
- Seated or standing calf raises: 3 sets of 12-15 repetitions

Flexibility (10 minutes)

- Chest stretch: Hold for 15-30 seconds
- Quadriceps stretch: Hold for 15-30 seconds each leg
- Side stretches: Hold for 15-30 seconds each side

Cool-Down (5 minutes)

- Gentle stretching and deep breathing

Day 6: Cardio and Balance

Warm-Up (5-10 minutes)

- Light jogging or marching in place

Cardio (30 minutes)

- Swimming or water aerobics (if accessible)

- Elliptical machine or light jogging

Balance (10 minutes)

- Balance board exercises: 3 sets of 12-15 repetitions
- Stability ball exercises (seated or standing): 3 sets of 12-15 repetitions

Cool-Down (5 minutes)

- Slow walking and deep breathing

Day 7: Active Recovery

Active Recovery (30-40 minutes)

- Gentle yoga or stretching
- Leisurely walking or swimming

Relaxation

- Deep breathing exercises or meditation for 10-15 minutes

Advanced Workout Plan

Day 1: High-Intensity Interval Training (HIIT) and Flexibility

Warm-Up (5-10 minutes)

- Light jogging or brisk walking
- Dynamic stretches: leg swings, arm circles, and torso twists

HIIT (20 minutes)

- 30 seconds of high-intensity exercise (e.g., jogging in place, jumping jacks, or burpees)
- 30 seconds of low-intensity exercise or rest
- Repeat for 20 minutes

Flexibility (10 minutes)

- Neck stretches: Hold for 15-30 seconds each side
- Shoulder stretches: Hold for 15-30 seconds each side
- Hamstring stretches: Hold for 15-30 seconds each leg
- Calf stretches: Hold for 15-30 seconds each leg

Cool-Down (5 minutes)

- Slow walking and deep breathing

Day 2: Advanced Strength Training and Balance

Warm-Up (5-10 minutes)

- Light jogging or gentle stretching

Strength Training (45 minutes)

- Squats with weights: 4 sets of 12-15 repetitions
- Push-ups (standard or decline): 4 sets of 12-15 repetitions
- Bent-over rows: 4 sets of 12-15 repetitions each side

- Walking lunges with weights: 4 sets of 12-15 repetitions each leg
- Dumbbell bicep curls: 4 sets of 12-15 repetitions
- Tricep dips: 4 sets of 12-15 repetitions

Balance (10 minutes)

- Single-leg squats: 3 sets of 10-12 repetitions each leg
- Standing on one leg with eyes closed: 3 sets of 20-30 seconds each leg

Cool-Down (5 minutes)

- Gentle stretching and deep breathing

Day 3: Cardio and Mobility

Warm-Up (5-10 minutes)

- Light jogging or marching in place

Cardio (45 minutes)

- Cycling on a stationary bike, elliptical machine, or running

Mobility (10 minutes)

- Cat-cow stretch: 1-2 minutes
- Hip flexor stretch: Hold for 15-30 seconds each side
- Ankle circles: 1-2 minutes

Cool-Down (5 minutes)

- Slow walking and deep breathing

Day 4: Active Recovery

Active Recovery (30-40 minutes)

- Gentle yoga or stretching

- Leisurely walking or swimming

Relaxation

- Deep breathing exercises or meditation for 10-15 minutes

Day 5: Advanced Strength Training and Flexibility

Warm-Up (5-10 minutes)

- Light jogging or gentle stretching

Strength Training (45 minutes)

- Deadlifts: 4 sets of 12-15 repetitions

- Overhead shoulder presses: 4 sets of 12-15 repetitions

- Seated rows with resistance bands: 4 sets of 12-15 repetitions

- Bulgarian split squats: 4 sets of 12-15 repetitions each leg

- Seated leg presses: 4 sets of 12-15 repetitions

- Calf raises with weights: 4 sets of 12-15 repetitions

Flexibility (10 minutes)

- Chest stretch: Hold for 15-30 seconds

- Quadriceps stretch: Hold for 15-30 seconds each leg
- Side stretches: Hold for 15-30 seconds each side

Cool-Down (5 minutes)

- Gentle stretching and deep breathing

Day 6: Cardio and Balance

Warm-Up (5-10 minutes)

- Light jogging or marching in place

Cardio (45 minutes)

- Swimming or water aerobics (if accessible)
- High-intensity interval training (HIIT) on an elliptical machine or treadmill

Balance (10 minutes)

- Balance board exercises: 3 sets of 12-15 repetitions
- Stability ball exercises (seated or standing): 3 sets of 12-15 repetitions

Cool-Down (5 minutes)

- Slow walking and deep breathing

Day 7: Active Recovery

Active Recovery (30-40 minutes)

- Gentle yoga or stretching
- Leisurely walking or swimming

Relaxation

- Deep breathing exercises or meditation for 10-15 minutes

Safety Tips and Injury Prevention

Before diving into specific safety tips, it's important to understand the common risks associated with exercise for seniors:

1. Joint Strain: Endomorphs may experience more stress on their joints due to higher body fat percentages.

2. Muscle Strain: Overexertion or improper form can lead to muscle strains.

3. Falls: Balance issues or slippery surfaces can increase the risk of falls.

4. Cardiovascular Events: Intense exercise can strain the heart, especially in those with pre-existing conditions.

General Safety Guidelines

1. Consult with Your Doctor:

- Medical Clearance: Before starting any new exercise program, consult your healthcare provider, especially if you have chronic conditions like arthritis, diabetes, or cardiovascular disease.

- Personalized Advice: Your doctor can provide tailored recommendations and highlight any specific exercises to avoid.

2. Start Slowly:

- Gradual Progression: Begin with low-intensity exercises and gradually increase the intensity and duration as your fitness improves.
- Warm-Up and Cool-Down: Always start with a warm-up to prepare your body for exercise and end with a cool-down to aid recovery.

3. Listen to Your Body:

- Pain vs. Discomfort: Understand the difference between discomfort, which can be normal, and pain, which can indicate injury. Stop exercising if you experience pain.
- Rest and Recovery: Allow adequate rest between workouts to prevent overtraining and give your muscles time to recover.

4. Stay Hydrated:

- Hydration: Drink plenty of water before, during, and after exercise to stay hydrated and maintain performance.
- Electrolytes: Consider electrolyte-rich drinks if you're engaging in prolonged or intense workouts.

Specific Injury Prevention Strategies

1. Proper Form and Technique:

- Learn Correct Form: Use proper form for all exercises to prevent strains and injuries. If unsure, consider working with a personal trainer.
- Avoid High-Impact Exercises: Opt for low-impact exercises like swimming, cycling, or walking to reduce stress on your joints.

2. Use Appropriate Equipment:

- Supportive Footwear: Wear shoes that provide good support and cushioning to protect your feet and joints.
- Adaptive Equipment: Use equipment like resistance bands, stability balls, and light weights that are appropriate for your fitness level.

3. Balance and Flexibility:

- Balance Exercises: Incorporate exercises that improve balance, such as tai chi, yoga, or standing on one leg.
- Stretching: Regularly stretch all major muscle groups to maintain flexibility and reduce the risk of muscle strains.

4. Strength Training:

- Low Weights, High Repetitions: Use lighter weights with higher repetitions to build strength without overloading your muscles and joints.
- Target Core Strength: Strengthen your core muscles to improve stability and reduce the risk of falls.

Environmental Considerations

1. Safe Environment:

- Clear Space: Ensure your workout area is free from obstacles that could cause trips or falls.
- Non-Slip Mats: Use non-slip mats for floor exercises to prevent slipping.

2. Temperature and Weather:

- Avoid Extreme Conditions: Exercise indoors during extreme weather conditions to avoid heat stroke, dehydration, or hypothermia.
- Dress Appropriately: Wear appropriate clothing for the weather, including layers in colder temperatures and breathable fabrics in the heat.

3. Proper Lighting:

- Well-Lit Areas: Ensure your workout space is well-lit to prevent accidents and improve visibility.

Monitoring Your Health

1. Heart Rate Monitoring:

- Heart Rate Zones: Use a heart rate monitor to ensure you're exercising within your target heart rate zone, especially during cardiovascular exercises.
- Regular Checks: Regularly check your heart rate and adjust your intensity as needed.

2. Signs of Overexertion:

- Breathlessness: If you're excessively breathless, slow down or take a break.

- Dizziness or Lightheadedness: Stop exercising and rest if you feel dizzy or lightheaded.

3. Regular Health Check-Ups:

- Routine Visits: Schedule regular check-ups with your healthcare provider to monitor your overall health and make necessary adjustments to your exercise routine.

Adapting to Your Body's Changes

1. Age-Related Adjustments:

- Modified Exercises: Modify exercises to accommodate any age-related changes in flexibility, strength, and endurance.
- Low-Impact Alternatives: Choose low-impact activities that are gentler on your joints.

2. Chronic Conditions:

- Special Considerations: If you have chronic conditions like arthritis, osteoporosis, or diabetes, follow specific exercise guidelines tailored to your condition.

- Medication Effects: Be aware of how your medications might affect your exercise tolerance and make adjustments accordingly.

Emergency Preparedness

1. Emergency Contacts:

- Contact Information: Keep a list of emergency contacts accessible during your workouts.
- Medical ID: Consider wearing a medical ID bracelet if you have significant health conditions.

2. First Aid Knowledge:

- Basic Skills: Learn basic first aid skills, including how to recognize and respond to signs of a heart attack or stroke.
- Emergency Plan: Have a plan in place for seeking help if an emergency arises during your workout.

Conclusion

As we conclude this comprehensive guide, it's clear that aging gracefully and maintaining optimal health as an endomorph senior is a multifaceted journey. By understanding your unique body type, you can tailor your approach to nutrition and exercise, ensuring that your efforts are both effective and sustainable. The knowledge and strategies provided throughout this book are designed to empower you to take control of your health and well-being, making informed decisions that support your fitness goals.

We've explored the fundamental characteristics of endomorph seniors, highlighting the importance of recognizing your body's natural tendencies. This understanding forms the foundation upon which you can build a personalized fitness and nutrition plan. Acknowledging the challenges and advantages of your body type enables you to approach your health journey with realistic expectations and a positive mindset.

Nutrition plays a pivotal role in the health of endomorph seniors. By focusing on balanced macronutrients and essential micronutrients, you can optimize your diet to support weight management, energy levels, and overall health. The detailed meal plans, shopping lists, and meal prep tips provided in this book serve as practical tools to help you implement these nutritional principles into your daily life. Remember, the key is to find a balance that works for you and to be consistent in your efforts.

Exercise is equally important in maintaining your health and vitality as an endomorph senior. Safe and effective workouts, whether performed at home or in the gym, are essential for building strength, improving cardiovascular health, and enhancing flexibility and mobility. The various workout plans and exercise tips outlined in this book are designed to cater to your fitness level and preferences, ensuring that you can stay active and motivated.

Injury prevention and safety are critical components of any fitness regimen, especially for seniors. By following the safety guidelines and injury prevention strategies discussed, you can reduce the risk of setbacks and continue to enjoy the benefits of regular physical activity. Prioritizing your safety and well-being will help you maintain a consistent and enjoyable exercise routine.

Ultimately, the journey to better health as an endomorph senior is a lifelong commitment. Embrace the process, celebrate your progress, and be patient with yourself as you navigate the challenges and triumphs along the way. With the knowledge and tools provided in this book, you are well-equipped to achieve your health and fitness goals, leading to a more vibrant, energetic, and fulfilling life. Remember, your health is your most valuable asset—nurture it with care and dedication.

www.ingramcontent.com/pod-product-compliance
Lightning Source LLC
Chambersburg PA
CBHW061511250726
48657CB00005B/1800